# Five-Minute
# Face-lift

# Five-Minute Face-lift

## A Daily Program for a Beautiful, Wrinkle-Free Face

Reinhold Benz

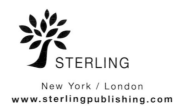

STERLING

New York / London
www.sterlingpublishing.com

STERLING and the distinctive Sterling logo are registered trademarks of
Sterling Publishing Co., Inc.

**Library of Congress Cataloging-in-Publication Data**

Benz, Reinhold.
 [Facebuilding. English]
 Facebuilding : the daily 5-minute program for a beautiful, wrinklefree face / Reinhold Benz.
      p. cm.
 Translation of: Facebuilding
 Includes index.
 ISBN 0-8069-8340-X. — ISBN 0-8069-8339-6 (pbk.)
 1. Beauty, Personal.   2. Face—Care and hygiene.   I. Title.
 RA778.B4713  1991
 646.7'26—dc20                                          90-24302
                                                        CIP

10  9  8  7  6  5  4  3  2

Published by Sterling Publishing Co., Inc.
387 Park Avenue South, New York, NY 10016
Original edition published under the title
*Facebuilding: Das tägliche 5-minuten-programm für
ein schönes und faltenfries gesicht* © 1990 by
Sunset Verlag, 8000 München 19
English translation © 1991 by Sterling Publishing Co., Inc.
Previously published under the title
*Facebuilding: The Daily 5-Minute Program for a Beautiful, Wrinkle-free Face*
Distributed in Canada by Sterling Publishing
<sup>c</sup>/o Canadian Manda Group, 165 Dufferin Street
Toronto, Ontario, Canada M6K 3H6
Distributed in the United Kingdom by GMC Distribution Services
Castle Place, 166 High Street, Lewes, East Sussex, England BN7 1XU
Distributed in Australia by Capricorn Link (Australia) Pty. Ltd.
P.O. Box 704, Windsor, NSW 2756, Australia

*Printed in China*
*All rights reserved*

Sterling ISBN-13: 978-1-4027-5372-5
        ISBN-10: 1-4027-5372-1

For information about custom editions, special sales, premium and
corporate purchases, please contact Sterling Special Sales
Department at 800-805-5489 or specialsales@sterlingpublishing.com.

# FOREWORD

No matter where I am, in my consultation room, in the halls of the clinic, even at home, not a day goes by without patients—women, and in increasing numbers men too—asking me for a natural remedy to combat wrinkles, a remedy without the scalpel or collagen injections. I am a plastic surgeon; don't I know something one can do as a preventative measure?

My replies always used to be general: sufficient sleep, correct nutrition, healthy life style, and the use of some cosmetics.

Cynics might interpret such advice as an admission of helplessness. After all, there is no such thing as a prevention against the natural process of aging. Or is there?

Then, I came across this book: attractive photos, interesting anatomical drawings; on the left side a drawing of the muscle, on the right the exercise; on the left anatomy, on the right the effect.

Here it was—the remedy. The author calls it "Facebuilding." He concentrates on twenty-one of the most important facial muscles—those that determine our facial expressions. Because they are not constantly used, moved, or trained, they lose suppleness, vitality, and elasticity and because skin and muscles are so closely connected, our face gets older, gets wrinkles.

As a bodybuilder trains his muscular body, a facebuilder trains his facial muscles. And the face remains young, supple, fresh, and the skin retains its elasticity. The effort: five to ten minutes a day, wherever you choose.

Werner L. Mang, M.D.
Clinic for Plastic and Aesthetic Surgery
Bodensee

# CONTENTS

# INTRODUCTION

# PREFACE

A few years ago I saw some wonderful photos of a prima ballerina in a magazine. She had a beautiful, firm, youthful body. It was faultless—a perfect example of a perfect body.

Her face, however, was in stark contrast to her beautiful body. It showed definite signs of aging. I later learned that the dancer was 42 years old, which explained why she did not have the face of a young woman. Nevertheless, I was surprised that a 42-year-old woman could have such a perfect, youthful body while her face showed all the signs of her age. How was that possible?

There could be only one explanation: As a dancer she was involved in continuous training and exercises; she had tight, well contoured muscles with a skin that had maintained a wonderful, youthful elasticity. But why didn't her face look as young and smooth as her body?

The answer wasn't hard to find: *The prima ballerina never exercised her face—only her body.*

The picture of the prima ballerina has stayed with me to this day. Frequently, my thoughts returned to those magazine photographs. Was it possible to train a face as one could a body? To preserve or regain the youthfulness that once was?

I knew it was possible with a body. Dancers and bodybuilding enthusiasts have proven it time and time again. But why have we never thought of training facial muscles? The idea of finding an answer was not to leave me.

I found many books about bodybuilding, but nothing on the subject of the training of facial muscles. It was clear to me: I was on my own. I initiated research on the subject, and in the course of a few years a whole new, revolutionary method, which I called *Face Building*, began to evolve.

# THE STRUCTURE UNDERLYING BEAUTY

Two anatomical structures supply the basic support for facial beauty: One is the facial musculature; the other is the subcutaneous tissue directly under the surface of the skin, which provides its elasticity. Facial muscles and facial skin are closely connected, which is why the skin is able to follow every movement of the muscles. But it is precisely this close a connection that causes the condition and structure of the muscles to have such an impact on how we look. If the muscle structures lose their strength, it is bound to affect the skin.

And the same holds true for the second facial structure: the tissue that gives the skin its elasticity and its smooth, youthful, and wrinkle-free appearance.

Skin will lose its elasticity whenever tissue fibre begins to atrophy (to atrophy means that the fibre is in the process of being reduced in volume).

This is precisely what happens during the aging process—muscle and tissue fibre literally decrease. The facial musculature and the subcutaneous tissue lose tone and volume.

This aging process, however, can be considerably slowed down if a training and exercise program, specifically geared to the facial muscles, is instituted. This means that, by undertaking a sensible exercise program of the facial musculature, the aging process can be slowed down and already existing "weak spots" can be totally—or in part—regenerated.

# WHAT IS FACEBUILDING?

Musculature and tissue increases in volume and tone when exercised.

Facebuilding is accomplished with a systematic training program, specifically designed to exercise facial musculature. It is important that exercises are carried out correctly and the program is adhered to as described. In other words, make sure that each step is performed with great care and attention.

Logic tells us that the aging process of the face can be slowed down and damage due to deterioration be reversed, either wholly or at least in part, because we have been successful in doing that—and for a long time—with our bodies.

The exercises that have been developed will effectively return weak muscles—that have turned into something resembling overstretched rubber bands—to a healthy, well-toned condition. As a matter of fact, the exercises will *prevent* healthy muscles from getting into such a sorry state.

In the course of the exercises the skin that covers facial musculature is gently stretched, something that happens naturally in reaction to the movements of muscles.

This gentle stretching is a physiological pro-

cess which will, in effect, increase and regenerate the production of collagen and elastin, two substances that are important for the elasticity of the skin.

Everyday, automatic movements of facial muscles are not sufficient to keep the elasticity of the fibres in good, firm, youthful condition. It is not beneficial *not* to exercise, on the contrary—the opposite is true. If the face is allowed to remain "unmoved," which is the natural state of affairs, muscles and tissues begin to atrophy and the result is loose, wrinkled skin that has taken on a "wilted" look.

Daily five-or ten-minute exercises, however, have an almost miraculous effect. After only two or three months you will be admired for your youthful, beautiful, clear, firm skin and the well-defined contours of your face.

Naturally, facebuilding exercises can also considerably postpone the aging process of the skin and even reverse it. It is not uncommon to be able to "turn back the clock" by as much as ten to fifteen years.

The facial exercises have another benefit: they increase blood circulation to the face, which in turn permits more oxygen and more nutrients to reach the cells of the skin. The cleansing process is equally as important and increased circulation considerably aids this process also. In addition, the ability of the skin to absorb moisture is increased.

An increased, internal availability of oxygen and good nutrition, with a simultaneous increase in effective cleansing of the tissues, is a sure guarantee for a clear, healthy skin without the unsightly enlargement of pores.

As important as the "internal care" is for your skin, do not forget to pamper it with appropriate, good cosmetic preparations.

# THE ADVANTAGES OF FACEBUILDING

1. Loose skin is "lifted": The skin regains a youthful, firm appearance.
2. The elasticity of the skin is improved: The skin is able to firmly and tightly cover the musculature and thereby smooth out those much feared wrinkles and crows' feet.
3. The skin is better nourished, with the pores unclogged, and better able to absorb moisture; this will increase and strengthen the fibre of the connective tissues and the skin will be firmer, large pores will be decreased, and the skin will regain a rosy, healthy, and firm appearance.

All are advantages that no woman wants to miss.

# HOW TO EXERCISE MOST EFFICIENTLY

Before starting on the exercise program, determine which of the facial features you are most concerned about. Use the guidelines in this book for choosing the exercises appropriate for the "problem zones." Note: You should do no more than five or six exercises.

I am sure that there are women who will tell me that they need each and every one of the exercises listed. All I can say is: First do those that you need most, because to do them all requires more time. But if you have the time, there is nothing wrong with doing them all.

Stand or sit in front of a mirror. The illustrations and photos show clearly which muscle you are working on for a particular exercise and in which direction the muscle fibre is running. Try to do the exercises as accurately as you can. Visualize the muscle. It might be helpful to put your fingers on the muscle so that you can "feel" in which direction the muscle fibres are moving and what it feels like when a muscle is exercised. *Every exercise should be performed with every ounce of energy that you can muster. The maximum tension should be held for at least six seconds.*

In the beginning, when the musculature is rather weak and loose, the maximum tension that you can create will not be very strong. The force of tension will increase, however, from week to week.

# HOW MUCH EXERCISE BEFORE RESULTS ARE NOTICEABLE?

The exercises have to be done regularly, at least five times a week. For the first two weeks, do each exercise five times. After two weeks increase each by five repetitions, for two more weeks, until twenty repetitions for each exercise have been reached.

Training will be at its most effective when you have reached twenty repetitions for each exercise, with no more than one-second intervals between each. But every one has to be executed with the maximum force. Also, it is not necessary to pause between exercises. The time needed for five to six exercises should be no more than five to ten minutes.

Visible changes can be expected after two or three months. Do not, therefore, expect miracles after two weeks. We know from various training programs for the body that it takes time to regenerate and rebuild the musculature.

It is important that you continue with your program once a satisfactory result has been obtained—although no more than two to three times a week is necessary.

# BASIC OBSERVATIONS CONCERNING THE POSITIONING OF HAND AND FINGERS

Placing fingers over the region to be exercised eliminates the possibility of creating artificial folds or wrinkles. But your fingers should touch the skin only lightly. Under no circumstances should the skin be stretched or pulled.

There are exercises that do not require the aid of fingers. If a fold or wrinkle seems to increase when doing that particular exercise, place one finger on the fold, anyway. This little trick will prevent artificial folds from being created.

# THE EXERCISES

## 1
# THE MUSCLE

# MUSCULUS FRONTALIS

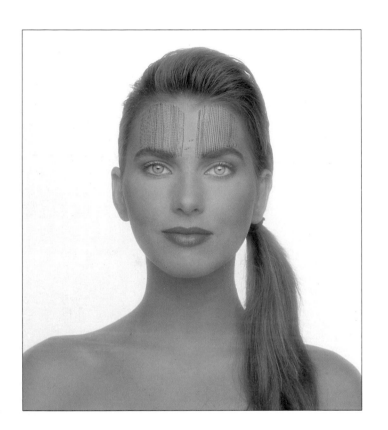
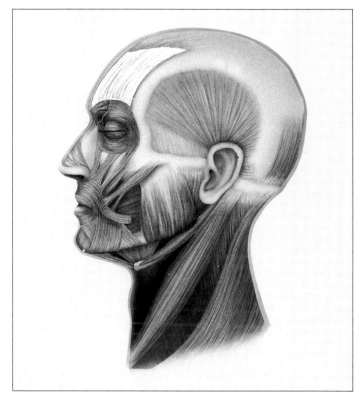

### SOURCE
The skin of the eyebrow

### START
At the forehead, reaching up to the hairline

### FUNCTION
The musculus frontalis lifts eyebrows and pulls the scalp forward. This action creates the wrinkles on the forehead.

18

# 1
# THE EXERCISE

## FOR A BEAUTIFUL FOREHEAD

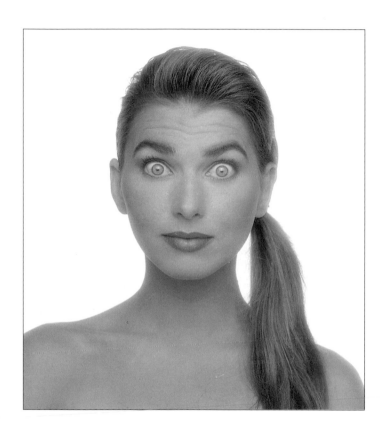 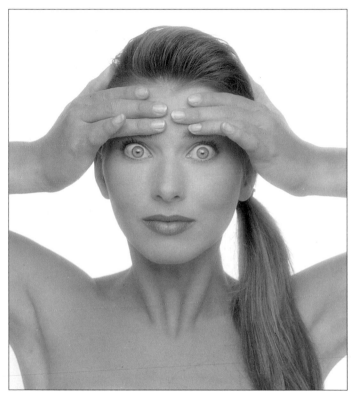

The left photo shows the exercise performed without the aid of your fingers and shows clearly an increase in the formation of the wrinkles on the forehead. In order to prevent that happening, put your fingers, as illustrated in the right photo, across the forehead so that both ring fingers rest comfortably across the eyebrows. Now try, against the pressure of your fingers, to lift your eyebrows and to pull the scalp forward.

# MUSCULUS TEMPORALIS

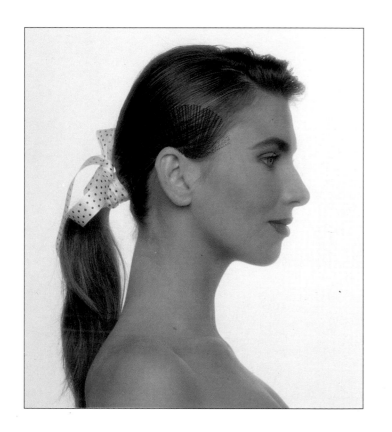
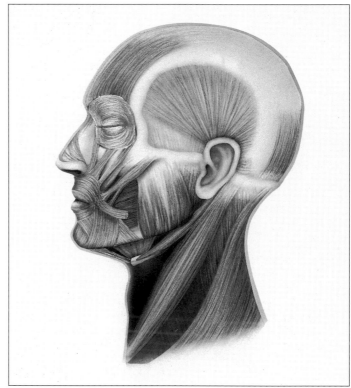

### SOURCE
Slightly above the ear

### START
At the temple region

### FUNCTION
Closes jaws and pulls back a lower protruding jaw

## 2
## THE EXERCISE

# FOR A BEAUTIFUL EYE-TEMPLE AREA

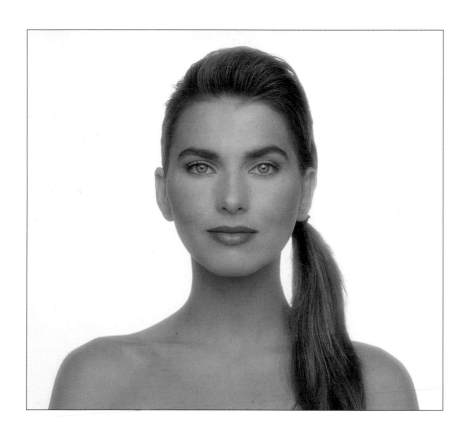

Pull your scalp back. Concentrate on, and visualize, the temple region. This exercise primarily trains the musculus occipitalis, but the musculus temporalis is automatically exercised throughout. If the exercise is performed correctly, the tension in that muscle will make the ears move backwards. The actual action, of course, is not visible in the photo.

If you have mastered the "ear movement," concentrate solely on your ears and the temple region. That will exercise the musculus temporalis. The training of the musculus temporalis is one of the most important exercises, because it will tighten and strengthen the whole upper portion of the face. A strong musculus temporalis will prevent crows'-feet.

# THE MUSCLE

## MUSCULUS CORRUGATOR GLABELLAE

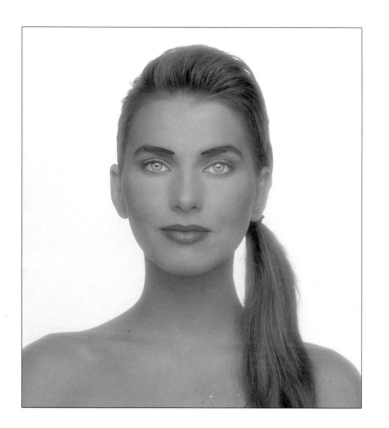 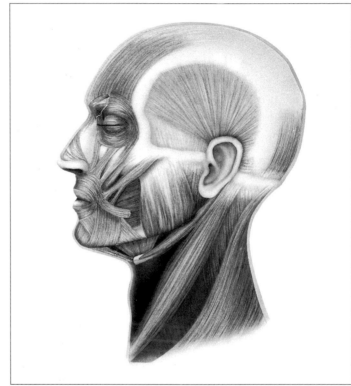

### SOURCE
From the nasal and frontal bone

### START
At the middle of the eyebrow

### FUNCTION
Frowning, causing a vertical fold at the top of the nose

# 3
# EXERCISE

## FOR NOSE AND FOREHEAD REGION

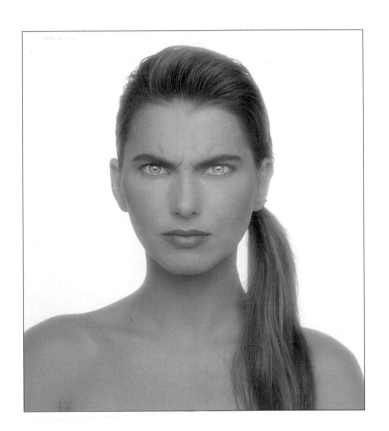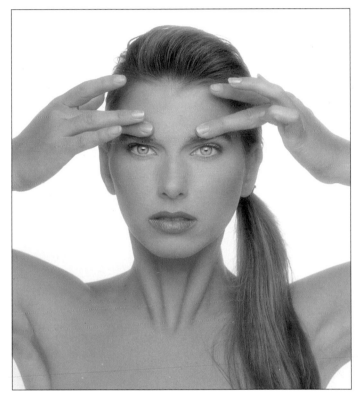

Pull eyebrows tightly together. Avoid the formation of a crease between the eyebrows by pressing with both index fingers lightly above the skin of both eyebrows, as shown.

# 4
# THE MUSCLE

## MUSCULUS ORBICULARIS OCCULI

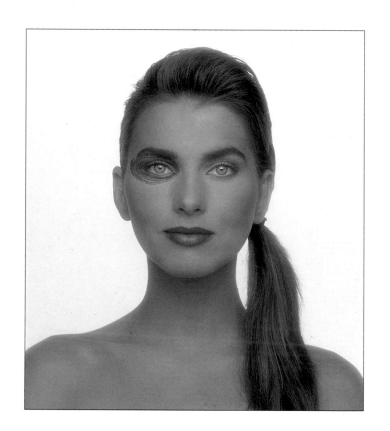

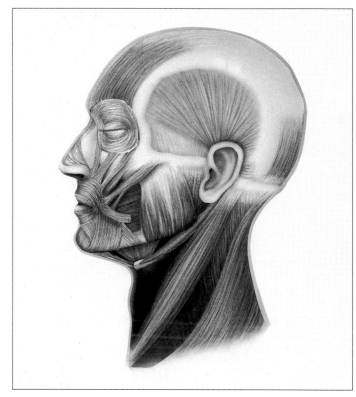

### SOURCE
The frontal bone and frontal-maxillary extension of the upper jaw to the inner lid

### START
A ring of muscles surrounding the orbital cavity in concentric circles

### FUNCTION
This muscle closes the eyes, pulls the eyebrows together and pulls the skin around the eye to the middle, which causes crows'-feet.

# 4
# THE EXERCISE

## TO BEAUTIFY THE AREA BELOW THE EYES

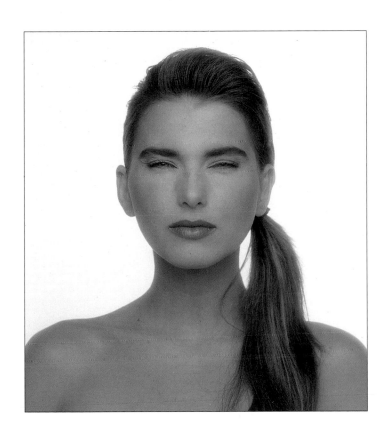 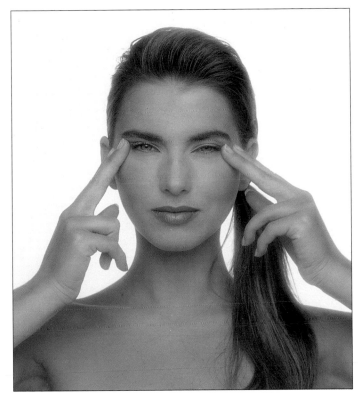

Keep your eyes open. Push lower lid up (left photo). The skin underneath and on both sides of the eyes will be pulled upwards and towards the nose (as if you were to look into the sun). To avoid wrinkling the skin, press it lightly with your fingers (see right photo).

# THE MUSCLE

## MUSCULUS ORBICULARIS OCCULI PARS PALEBRAL

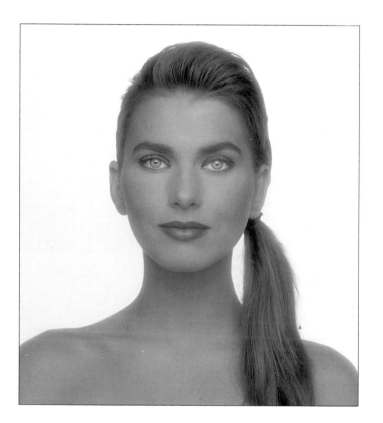

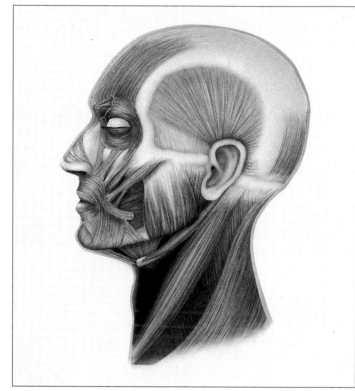

### SOURCE
From inside the lids

### START
The outer eyelid

### FUNCTION
To tightly close eyelids

# 5
# THE EXERCISE

## FOR A WRINKLE-FREE UPPER EYELID

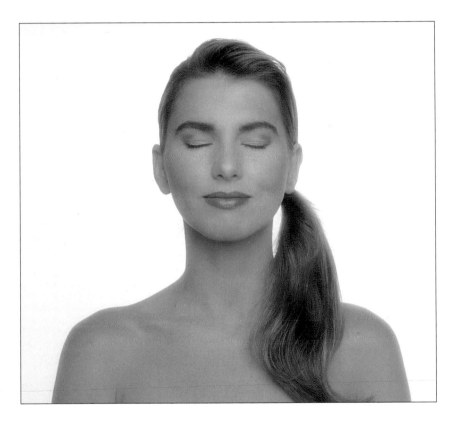

Close your eyes and press the upper lid down towards the lower lid.

# MUSCULUS LEVATOR PALPEBRAE SUPERIORS

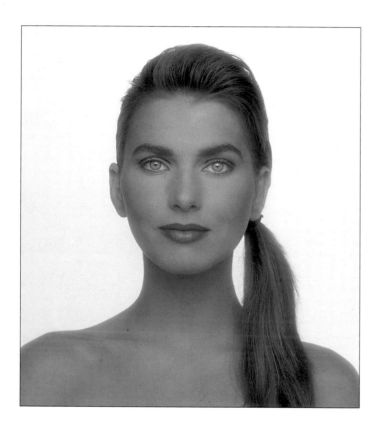
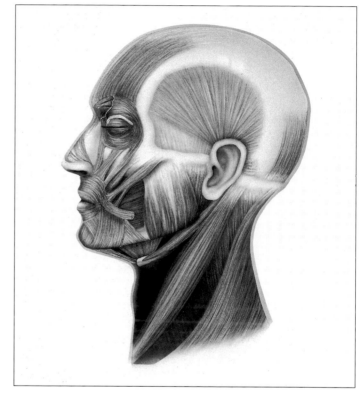

### SOURCE
The upper orbital rim

### START
The upper eyelid

### FUNCTION
To totally lift the upper lid

# 6
# THE EXERCISE

## TO PREVENT DROOPING UPPER EYELID

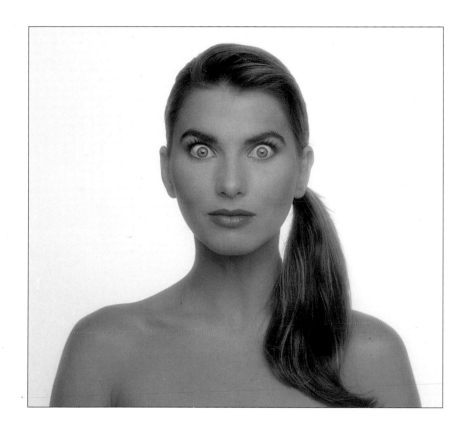

Pull upper lid upwards as far as possible with both eyes open. Make sure that the upper lid is pulled up until the white above the iris is visible.

# 7
# THE MUSCLE

## MUSCULUS ORBICULARIS OCCULI

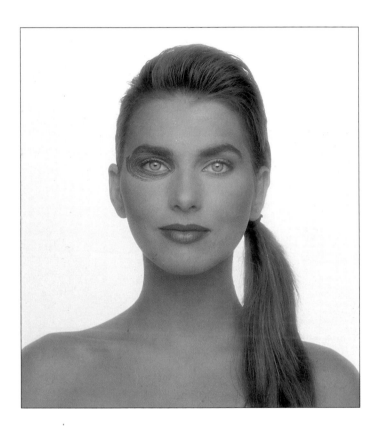
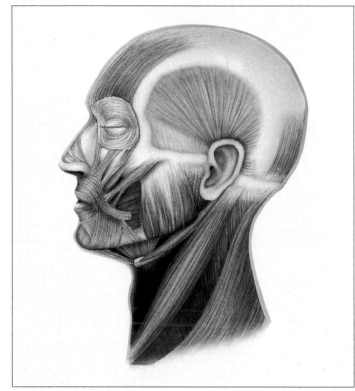

### SOURCE
The frontal bone and frontal-maxillary extension of the upper jaw to the ligaments of the inner lid

### START
A ring of muscles surrounding the orbital cavity in concentric circles

### FUNCTION
This muscle closes the eye and pulls the eyebrow down. Also, it pulls the skin around the eye towards the middle, creating crows'-feet

# 7
# THE EXERCISE

## TO BANISH CROW'S-FEET

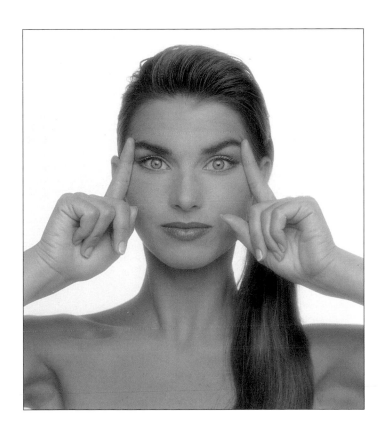 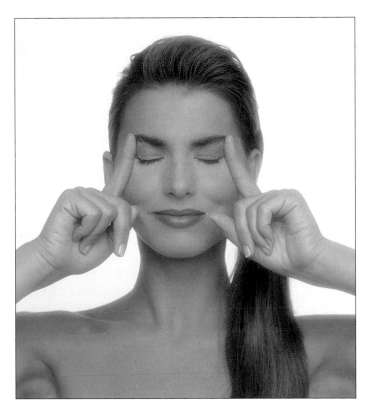

Position your fingers at the outer edge of the orbital cavity and close your eyes. The fingers are automatically pulled to the middle. Do not work against the movement of the muscle.

# 8
# THE MUSCLE

## MUSCULUS LEVATOR LABII SUPERIORIS

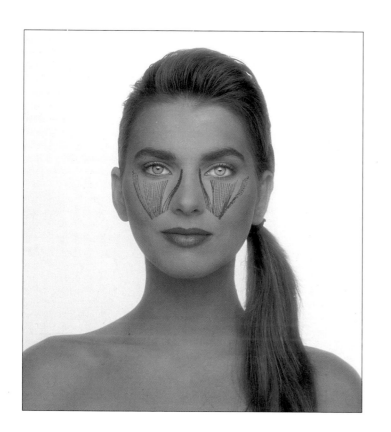

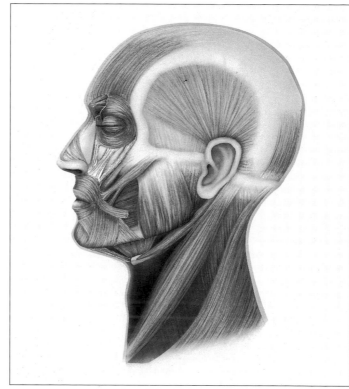

### SOURCE
The inner and outer rim of the orbital cavity

### START
The nose-lip indentation (see diagram in left photo)

### FUNCTION
To raise the upper lip

# 8
# THE EXERCISE

## FOR A BEAUTIFUL BLENDING FROM NOSE TO CHEEK

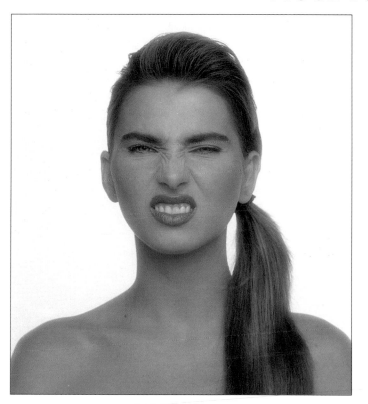 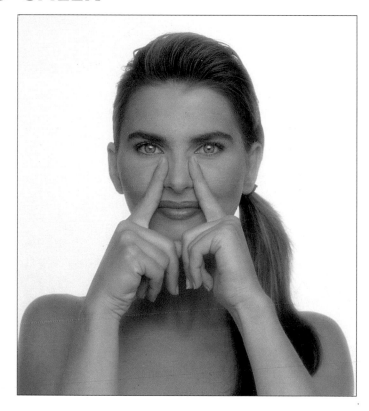

Flare your nostrils while wrinkling your nose. To prevent folds from forming, position your index, or middle, finger, as shown, from the inside of your eyes down to the corners of your mouth. The finger pressure will prevent the muscle from moving and thereby create an isometric form of exercise.

# 9
# THE MUSCLE

## MUSCULUS ZYGOMATICUS MAYOR

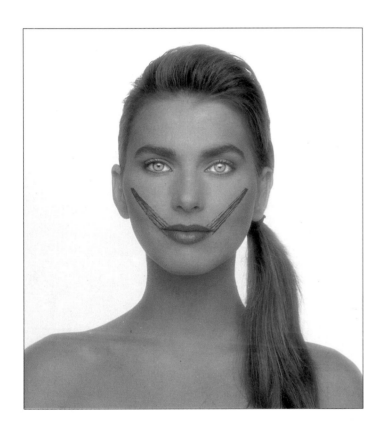
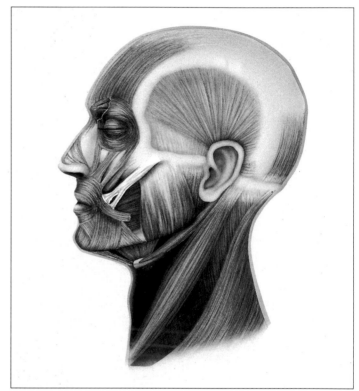

### SOURCE
The side of the cheekbone

### START
The corners of the mouth

### FUNCTION
Lifting the corners of the mouth to smile

# 9
# THE EXERCISE

## FOR A FIRM UPPER CHEEK AND UPWARDS-POINTING CORNERS OF THE MOUTH

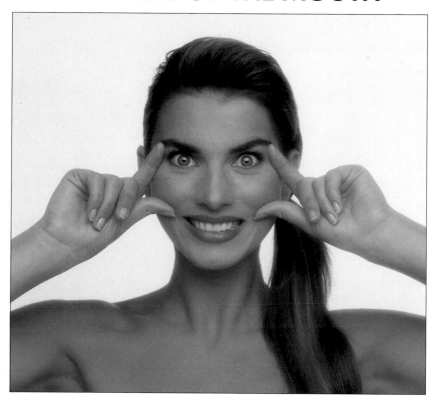

Pull the corners of your mouth up towards the outer cheekbone (as if laughing out loud), hold for approximately 6 seconds and release. In order not to create folds and wrinkles, put your index fingers next to the orbital cavity, as shown, and slightly touch the labial-nasal fold.

# 10
# THE MUSCLE

## MUSCULUS LEVATOR ANGULI ORIS
## (OR CANINUS)

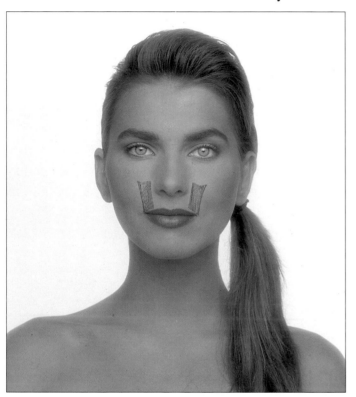 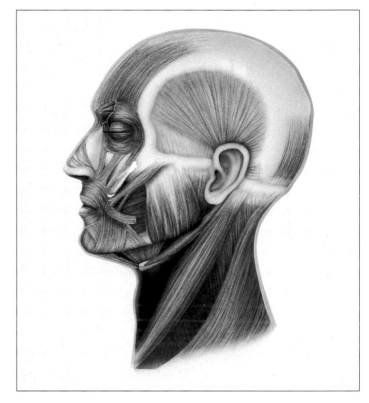

### SOURCE
Immediately under the lower medial rim of the
orbital cavity

### START
The corner of the mouth

### FUNCTION
Lifting the corner of the mouth

# 10
# THE EXERCISE

## TO LIFT THE CORNERS OF THE MOUTH

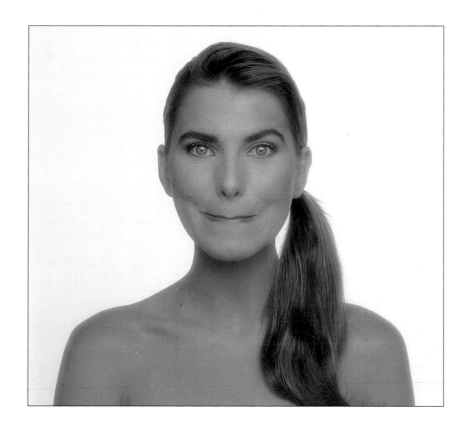

Pull your lips over your teeth. From this position, pull up both corners of the mouth.

# 11
# THE MUSCLE

# MUSCULUS RISORIUS

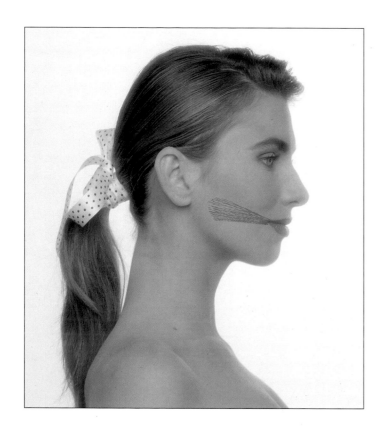
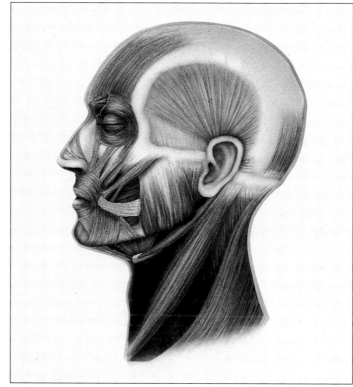

## SOURCE
The fascia of the masticatory muscle

## START
The corners of the mouth

## FUNCTION
Pulling the corners of the mouth sideways (when laughing, for example)

# 11
# THE EXERCISE

## FIRMING THE CHEEKS

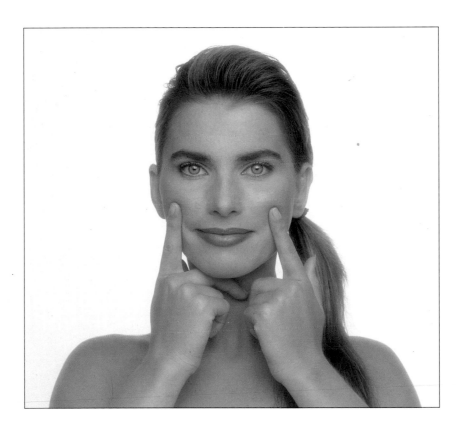

Pull the corners of your mouth to the outside. To avoid forming folds, put your index fingers to the corners of your mouth next to the nose-cheek fold.

# MUSCULUS BUCCINATOR

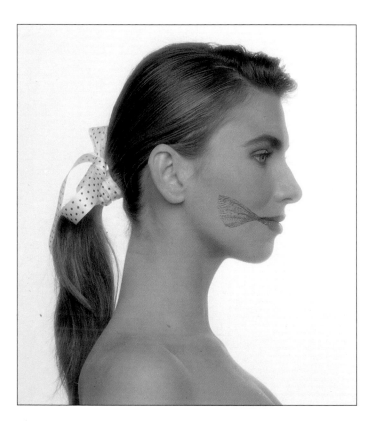
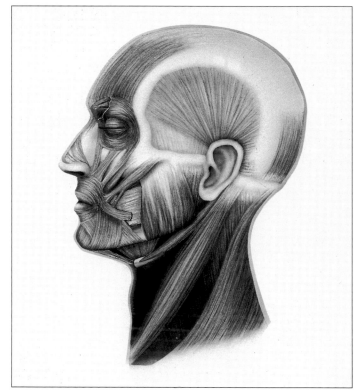

### SOURCE
The inside of the lower jaw

### START
The corner of the mouth

### FUNCTION
This muscle pushes the cheeks against the teeth.

## 12
## THE EXERCISE

# FIRMING LOWER CHEEK REGION

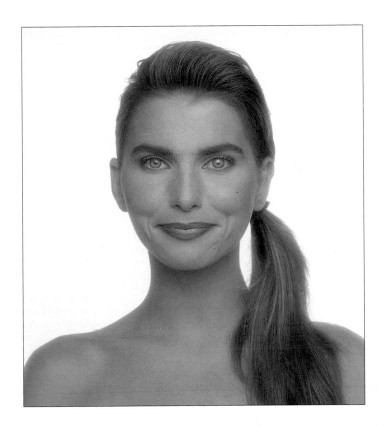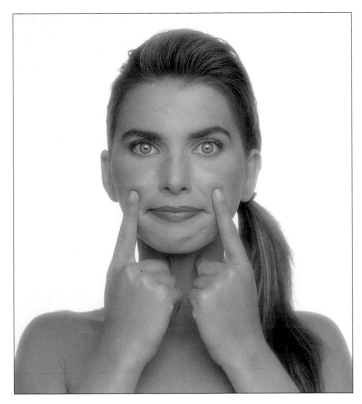

Close your lips, press cheek muscles to your teeth. To avoid creating wrinkles, lightly pull both corners of your mouth to the outside as shown.

# MUSCULUS ORBICULARIS ORIS

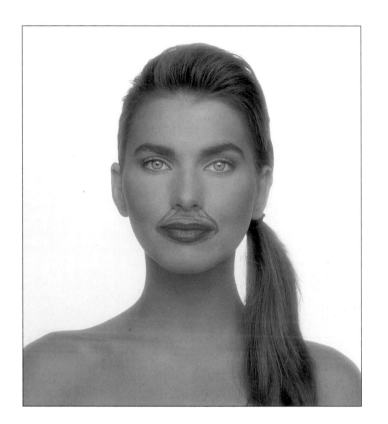

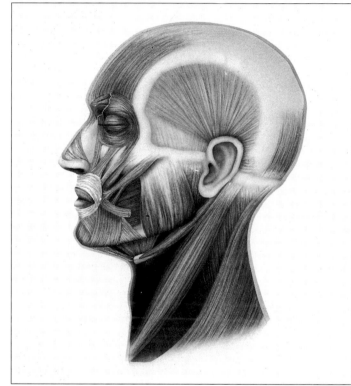

## SOURCE

This muscle consists of the sinewy fibres of the corners
of the mouth.

## START

Above the upper and below the lower lip (see diagram)

## FUNCTION

The muscles provide the basis for the structure of the
lips and function as the opening-and-closing mechanism
of the mouth.

# 13
# THE EXERCISE

# TO CREATE SMOOTH, BEAUTIFUL, FULL LIPS

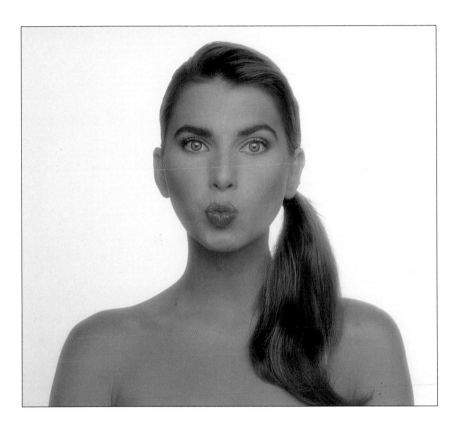

With forceful tension, pucker your lips, as if getting ready for a kiss (support the exercise by tightly pressing your nostrils together).

## 14
## THE MUSCLE

# MUSCULUS ORBICULARIS ORIS

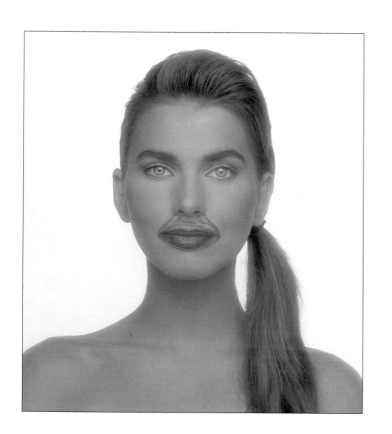

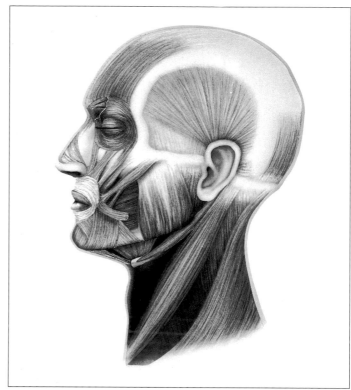

## SOURCE

This muscle consists of the sinewy fibres from the corners of the mouth.

## START

Above the upper and below the lower lip (see diagram)

## FUNCTION

The muscles provide the basis for the structure of the lips and function as the opening-and-closing mechanism of the mouth.

# 14
# THE EXERCISE

## TO CREATE FULL LIPS

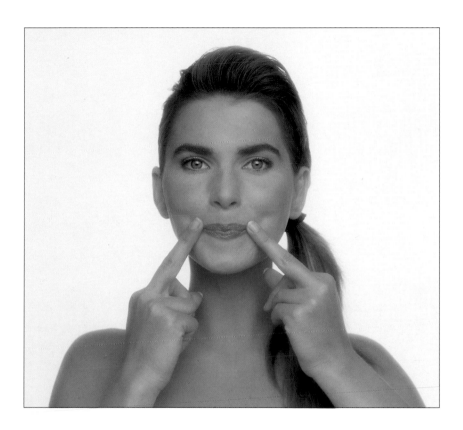

Press your lips tightly together. To avoid creating wrinkles, position the tip of your middle fingers at the corners of your mouth and pull slightly to the outside.

## 15
## THE MUSCLE

# MUSCULUS MENTALIS

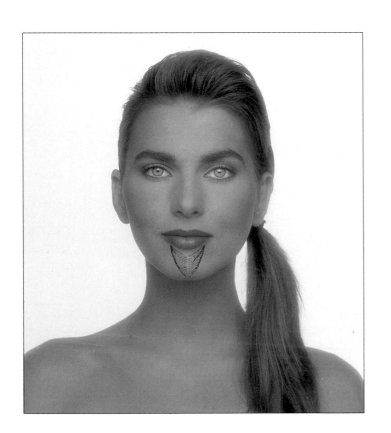

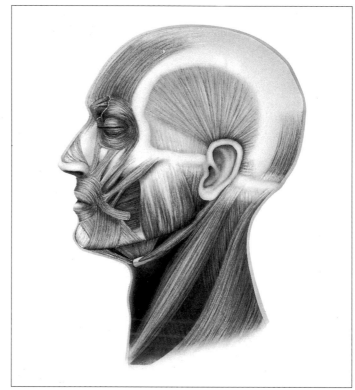

## SOURCE
The triangle between both canines

## START
The fibre tissue at the center of the chin

## FUNCTION
Pulling skin and tissue upwards

# TO CREATE A WELL FORMED CHIN

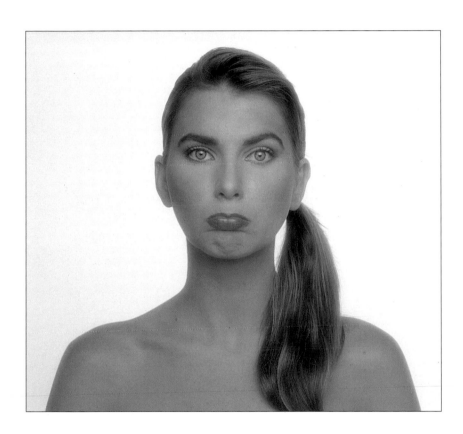

Pull the middle portion of your chin upwards to your lower lip. You should look as if you are pouting.

# 16
# THE MUSCLE

## MUSCULUS DEPRESSOR LABII INFERIORIS

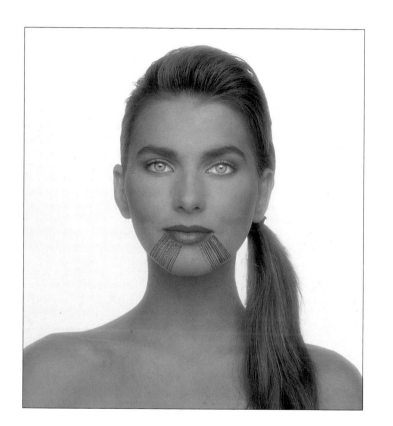
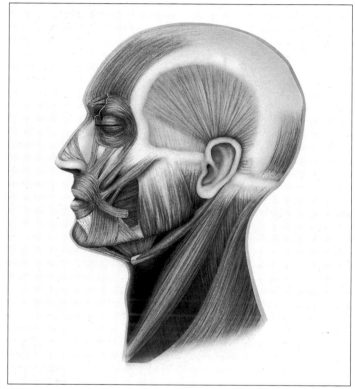

### SOURCE
The anterior section of the lower jawbone

### START
Extending from the base to both sides of the lower lip

### FUNCTION
Pushing the lower lip down

## 16
## THE EXERCISE

# TO CREATE A WELL CONTOURED CHIN

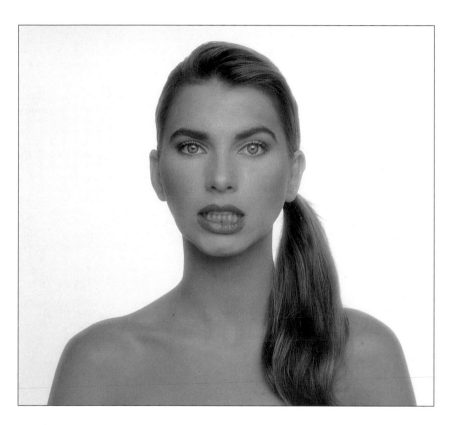

Push your lower lip down, until you can see your lower front teeth.
(Do not pull down the corners of your mouth.)

# MUSCULUS DEPRESSOR ANGULI ORIS

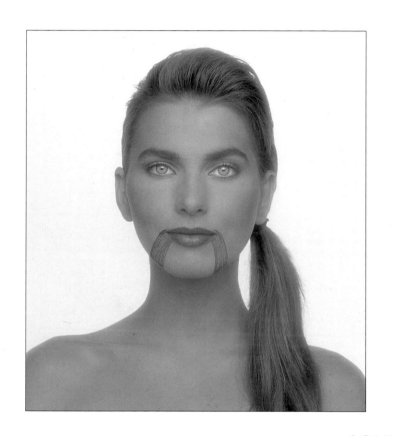
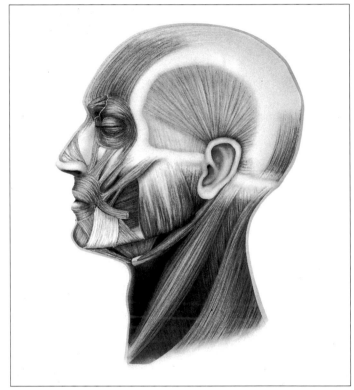

## SOURCE
The bony ridge at the edge of the lower jaw

## START
The corners of the mouth

## FUNCTION
Pushing down the corners of the mouth

# TO CREATE A WELL FORMED CHIN

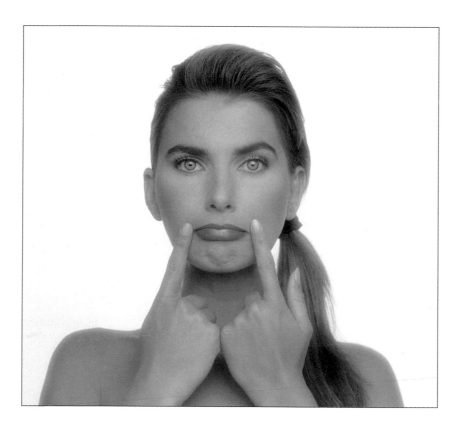

Push down the corners of your mouth. Keeping your index fingers lightly at the outside of the corners of the mouth will keep the skin from forming wrinkles.

# MUSCULUS PLATYSMA

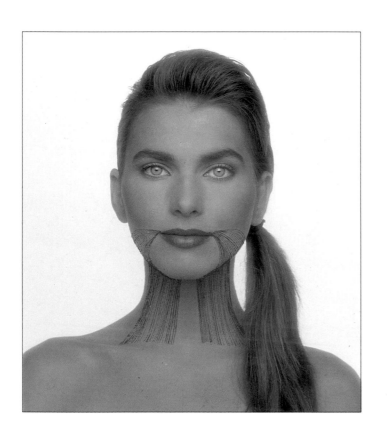
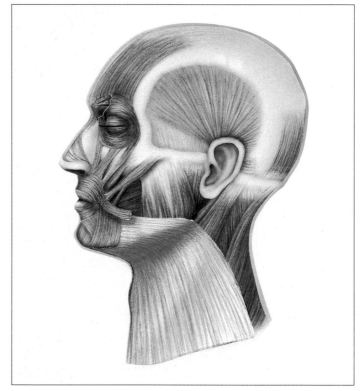

### SOURCE
The lower jaw and the corners of the mouth

### START
The fascia of the chest muscles

### FUNCTION
To tighten the skin at the neck

# 18
# THE EXERCISE

# TO FIRM UP THE AREA OF THE CHIN AND NECK

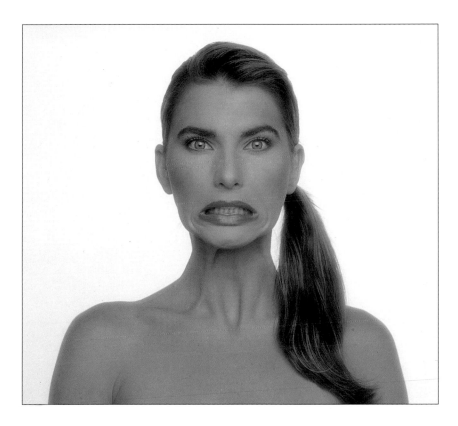

Tense the musculus platysma. This exercise is greatly supported if you forcefully pull down the lower lip, as shown. Correctly executed, the neck muscle will be clearly visible.

# MUSCULUS DIGASTRICUS

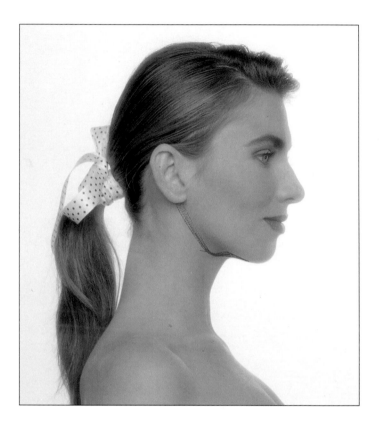
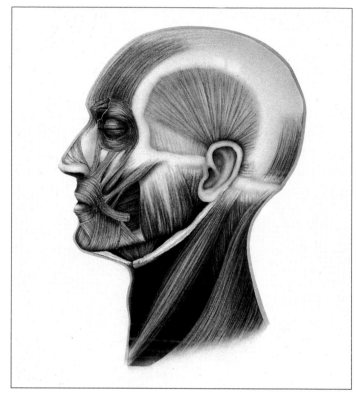

## SOURCE
The front portion at the inside of the lower jaw and the
back portion, behind the ear

## START
The tongue

## FUNCTION
Lowering lower jaw and lifting the tongue bone

# 19
# THE EXERCISE

## TO PREVENT A DOUBLE CHIN

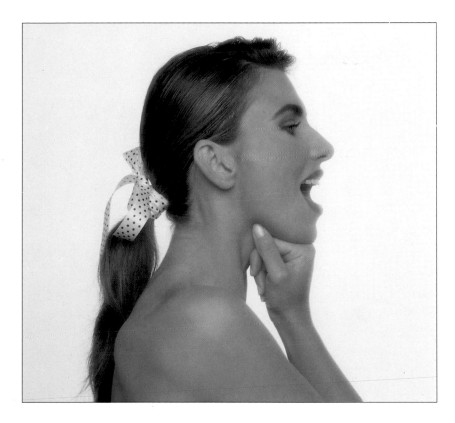

Position your hand under your chin, as shown in the photo above. Now force lower jaw open against the push of the fist.

# MUSCULUS MYLOHYOIDEUS

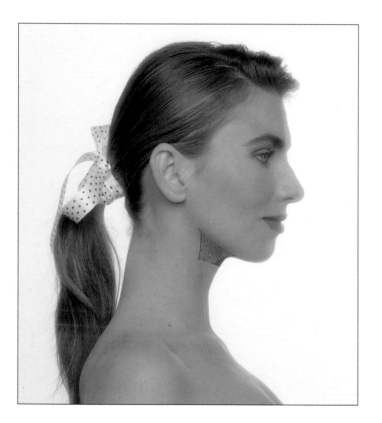
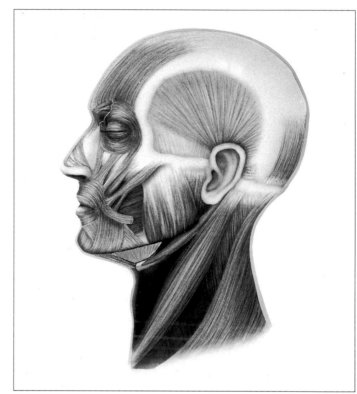

## SOURCE

The inside of the lower jaw

## START

The tongue

## FUNCTION

To lift tongue and tongue bone and to open lower jaw

# ELIMINATING OR REDUCING DOUBLE CHIN

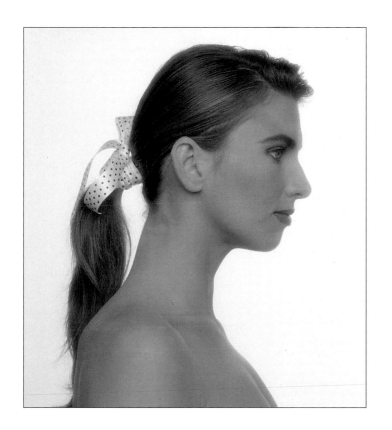 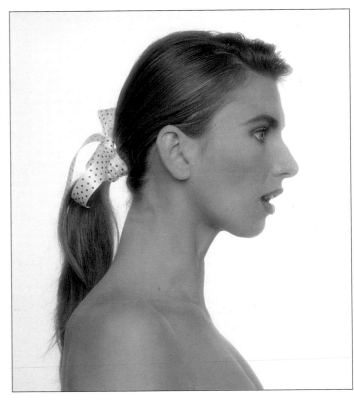

Press tongue against the roof of your mouth. Left photo was taken without muscle action. Right photo shows what the chin region will look like when muscle tension is activated.

# MUSCULUS MYLOHYOIDEUS

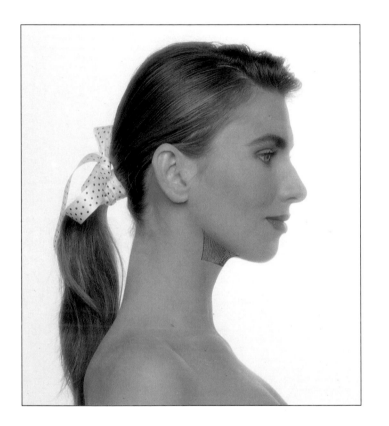 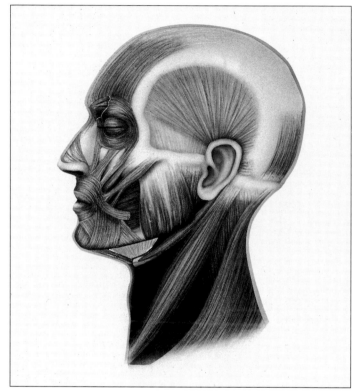

## SOURCE

The inside of the lower jaw

## START

The tongue

## FUNCTION

To lift tongue and tongue bone, and to open lower jaw

# 21
# THE EXERCISE

# TO PREVENT A DOUBLE CHIN

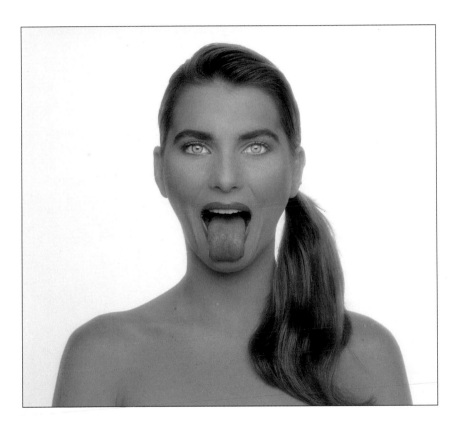

Stick out your tongue as shown in the photo above, and do it with as much force as you can muster.

# INDEX

Orbicularis oris, 42, 44
Origins of facebuilding, 12

## P

Platysma, 52
Positioning, hand and finger, 15, 19
Preventative exercise, 13
Problem zones, selection of, 15

## Q

Quantity of exercise, 15

## R

Reversing the aging process, 13
Risorius, 38

## S

Skin
   aging, 13
   elasticity improved, 13, 14
   loose lifted, 14
   pores unclogged, 14
Subcutaneous tissue, 12

## T

Temporalis, 20

## Z

Zygomaticus mayor, 34